Sleep

Discover How To Fall Asleep Easier, Get A Better Night's Rest, & Wake Up Feeling Energized

By Ace McCloud

Copyright © 2015

Disclaimer

The information provided in this book is designed to provide helpful information on the subjects discussed. This book is not meant to be used, nor should it be used, to diagnose or treat any medical condition. For diagnosis or treatment of any medical problem, consult your own physician. The publisher and author are not responsible for any specific health or allergy needs that may require medical supervision and are not liable for any damages or negative consequences from any treatment, action, application or preparation, to any person reading or following the information in this book. Any references included are provided for informational purposes only. Readers should be aware that any websites or links listed in this book may change.

Table of Contents

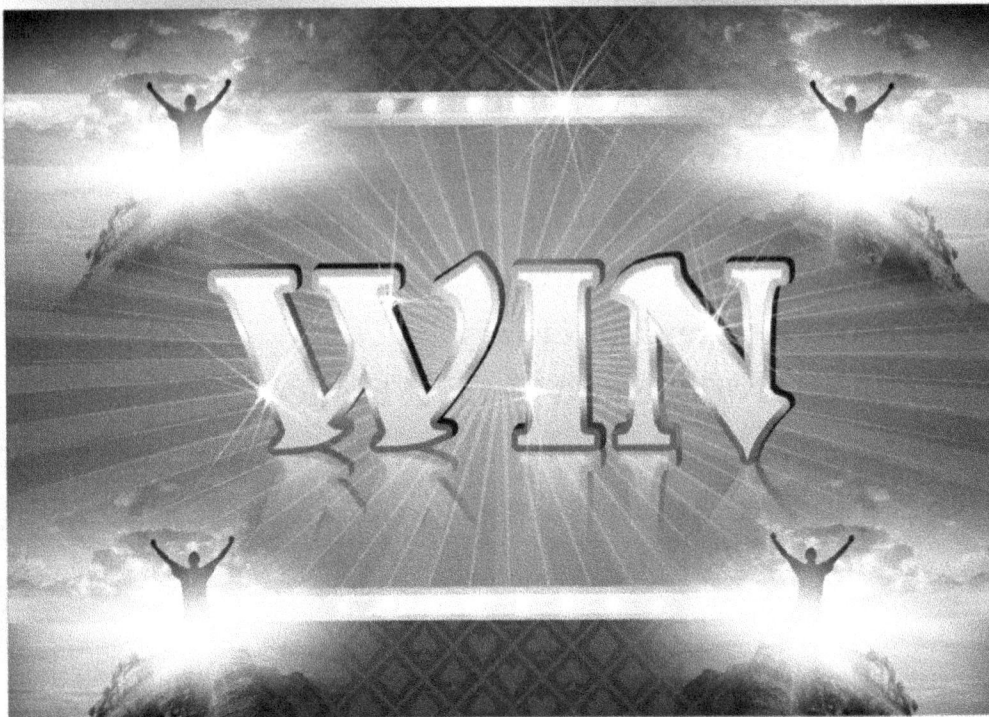

DEDICATED TO THOSE WHO ARE PLAYING THE GAME OF LIFE TO

WIN

KEEP ON PUSHING AND NEVER GIVE UP!

Ace McCloud

Be sure to check out my website for all my Books and Audio books.

www.AcesEbooks.com

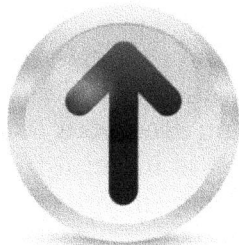

Introduction

I want to thank you and congratulate you for buying this book, "Sleep: Discover How To Fall Asleep Easier, Get A Better Nights Rest & Wake Up Feeling Energized"

This book contains proven steps and strategies on how to finally get the sleep you desperately need. We all require adequate sleep; if you are not getting enough of it on a regular basis, read on. You are about to take a journey that will improve your health and happiness. Sleep is integral to maintaining a number of bodily functions, so if you are not sleeping well, you cannot function normally.

The Centers for Disease Control and Prevention (CDC) say that lack of sleep is currently a major public health epidemic. According to recent reports approximately forty-eight percent of the people in the United States have stated that they do not sleep enough every day. A staggering seventy million people in the United States either suffer from wakefulness or a diagnosed sleeping disorder. Insomnia is a major cause of lack of sleep and it affects approximately one in three adults throughout the country. As you can see, if you are not sleeping, you are surely not alone.

While you sleep, your body goes to work to ensure that you are as healthy as possible. The cells in your body work to repair themselves, important hormones get released, and your brain gets a chance to recharge. Without these vital benefits, you are unable to fully function during the day.

The key is in knowing *how* to sleep well and for the right amount of time. Of course, this is easier said than actually accomplished for most people. It involves understanding your sleeping habits and working to replace the habits that stop you from catching enough Z's.

This book begins by explaining sleep. You will read the processes your body begins when your head hits the pillow. You will also discover how much sleep you actually need. While it is important to get enough sleep, oversleeping can be just as detrimental to your health as sleep deprivation.

You will learn what happens if you do not get adequate sleep. Missing out on sleep entirely for ten straight days can be fatal, which only underscores the how critical sleep is to your physical, mental, and emotional health. In this book, you will discover what happens when you are short on sleep and learn to identify the early warning signs that indicate you need to get more shuteye.

Since sleeping problems are increasingly common, you will learn here about various sleep disorders, how they are diagnosed, and what medical treatments are available. If you suspect you have a sleeping disorder, this book will help you both understand the disorder and speak knowledgeably with your doctor.

After you have a better understanding of what happens during sleep and what can cause problems, we will discuss what you can do throughout your day to improve your sleep. While it may sound strange, the things you do during the day have an impact on your ability to sleep at night.

There are times when, even though you have slept enough, you are still a little low on energy first thing in the morning. This book will suggest some strategies you can implement to boost your energy so that you awake refreshed and able to take on life's challenges.

A good night's sleep is partially dependent upon where you sleep and what you surround yourself with at night. You will learn what you can do to ensure that your bedroom is the perfect place to get a restful night's sleep. Follow the suggestions in these chapters to create a comfortable sleep sanctuary in which to dream the night away.

Few people are even aware that there is such a thing as sleep hygiene. In this book you will learn what it is and how to improve yours.

Finally, you will learn about creating an effective sleep routine and various natural remedies you can use to promote sleep.

Once you complete this book, you should be able to manage your sleep to improve your health, happiness, and your chances for success. If you implement the strategies described here, you may well find yourself better able to quickly solve problems and tackle your daily routine with vigor, due to the energy you will gain from sleeping so well. Welcome to this new journey and prepare to start experiencing the best sleep of your.

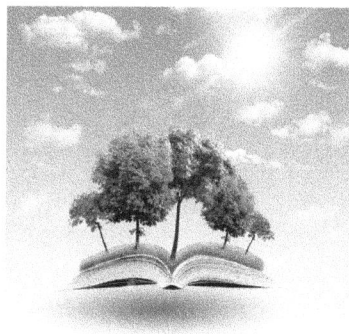

Chapter 1: How We Sleep

Sleep is a complex process that happens in four stages that are on a continuous cycle. Ideally, adults spend approximately one third of their day sleeping, so you want to get everything you can out of your down time. Did you know that not getting enough sleep can impair you just like alcohol can? This means that lack of sleep can make it dangerous to drive, hard to make decisions and difficult to tackle even simple tasks.

To best understand what is happening when you sleep, you need to understand the stages of sleep and what happens during each one.

Stage 1 Sleep: The first stage occurs approximately five to ten minutes after you fall asleep. Your muscles begin to relax, but you will wake easily if something disturbs you. A sudden muscle twitch during this stage can easily wake you up. Some people also encounter a falling sensation during this stage. In stage one you experience a very light sleep where you hover between sleep and wakefulness.

Stage 2 Sleep: The second stage of sleep covers approximately forty-five to fifty minutes. If you are awakened during this stage, you will experience disorientation. Your heart has an easier job since quite a few bodily processes slow down. Your body prepares for the next stage of sleep by reducing the activity of your brain and the interactions of the entire nervous system. In this stage you will experience:

- The onset of the sleep cycle

- A decreased awareness of your surroundings

- A lower body temperature

- No change in your heart rate or your breathing

Stage 3 Sleep: For about twenty minutes, your body rests in a deep sleep. Your brain emits steady and slow brain waves and your body uses the down time to begin the process of restoration. Substances that have accumulated in the brain throughout the day are flushed away. If you walk or talk in your sleep, this is when you will do so. At the same time, it is incredibly difficult to wake you during this stage of sleep.

Stage 4 Sleep: You are still sleeping deeply, but your brain is busy generating what scientists have labeled delta waves. No muscle activity or eye movement occurs during this stage. If you are wakened at this time, you will feel disoriented. This is the stage when children are most likely to experience night terrors, bedwetting, and sleepwalking.

Stages three and four share the same primary characteristics:

- You are in your deepest sleep.

- Your body is occupied with restoring, refreshing, and replenishing your cells.

- Your breathing is slowed.

- There is an increase in blood flow to your muscles.

- Your blood pressure is decreased.

- Your muscles are relaxed.

- Hormones are released into your body.

- Your energy is built up.

REM Sleep

Approximately ninety minutes after you fall asleep, you experience the first cycle of REM sleep. REM sleep, so named for the rapid eye movements that characterize this stage, will recur around every ninety minutes until you wake up.

While you are in REM sleep:

- Your eyes move back and forth.

- Your body and brain are fed energy.

- The increased brain activity triggers the presence of dreams.

- Your muscles are essentially turned off, leaving the body relaxed and immobile (except for your eyes, of course).

- Cortisol levels decrease.

- Procedural and spatial memory is stabilized within your brain.

- There is evidence that this sleep stage is critical for infant brain development

At its onset, some of the neurons in your brain stem are stimulated into activity, initiating the REM phase. During this stage, your brain stops producing monoamines – the neurotransmitters serotonin, dopamine, and noradrenaline.

Because your nerves are no longer transmitting instructions to your muscles, your body actually slips into a temporary paralysis.

This paralysis probably sounds scary, but it is necessary for full restoration during sleep. Those who do not experience the muscle paralysis may have a condition called REM behavior disorder, a condition that can cause someone to dramatically or violently act out their dreams.

As you get older, you typically need less REM sleep to feel rested. Scientists are still trying to determine exactly why this happens and if fewer REM cycles during sleep play a part in the degenerative aging of older adults.

How Much Sleep Do I Need?

Now that you know what happens while you sleep, it would help to understand how much sleep you need. Sleep requirements are different, depending on your age. The following are general recommendations for the minimum hours of sleep people need each night:

- Babies need at least sixteen hours of sleep.

- Children three to twelve years old need at least ten hours of sleep.

- Teenagers up to age eighteen also require at least ten hours of sleep.

- Adults aged nineteen to sixty-five need at least eight hours of sleep.

- Older adults beyond age sixty-five should have a minimum of six hours of sleep.

It is critical that you adhere to these guidelines on a regular basis. While oversleeping has its problems, getting too little sleep, even once a week, can engender potentially life-threatening situations. Your body requires adequate sleep on a daily basis, since it needs to be fully restored every twenty-four hours.

Benefits of Adequate Sleep

When you receive the amount of sleep your body needs, you are maximizing your chances for health in multiple aspects of your life. Here are a few ways that adequate sleep habits can allow your body to function at the peak of its ability:

Mental Wellbeing: Anxiety and depression are not uncommon among people who are exhausted. However, adequate sleep can maximize emotional stability and equip your mind and body to appropriately endure trials and tribulations when they do occur.

Healthy Marriage: Spending time together is important for increasing and strengthening the marital bond. However, many married couples are so exhausted that they do not spend quality time together. Adequate sleep can give you the energy you need to discuss important issues and make plans together as well as letting you enjoy a healthy libido.

Reduction of Pain: Whether you are experiencing an acute pain-generating injury or you are a chronic pain sufferer, it is important to seek adequate sleep. Getting enough sleep is critical to allow your body to heal itself, provide maximum circulation for healing medicines, and to help your body tolerate the trauma that is caused by the pain itself.

Clear Thinking: When you get enough sleep, you stand the greatest possible chance of thinking clearly, appropriately analyzing situations, and making sound decisions.

Reduced Injury Risk: When you are well-rested, there is a smaller chance of getting injured. This may sound obvious, since we just discussed mental clarity above. However, not only are your senses alert and able to identify potential dangers to avoid, your body is also better able to respond and correct your motion in order to prevent or minimize injury.

Maintain a Healthy Weight: People who get enough sleep are more likely to have and maintain healthy weight and fitness levels. Living at a healthy weight level will in turn allow and encourage the levels of physical of activity that are essential to optimal functioning of the entire person.

Fewer Episodes of Illness: When you consistently give yourself the sleep you need, your body will be equipped to fight off the normal bugs that infest your environment. Fewer illnesses translate into more days that are enjoyable, including undistracted time with loved ones as well as easier productivity at work.

Longer Life: You can increase your lifespan by getting enough sleep every night. Scientists are still trying to determine how this works. However, since sleep is critical to your overall health, it is not a great leap to say that getting adequate sleep can lengthen your life.

Decreased Inflammation: Inflammation is responsible for everything from diabetes, to premature aging, to pain and heart disease. Keeping inflammation under control is critical for a number of health processes. Research shows that inflammation is common among people who suffer from sleep apnea; however, when their apnea is under control, i. e. , they are getting adequate sleep, the blood work from these individuals indicates their inflammation is drastically reduced.

Maximized Creativity Getting enough sleep will allow you to work from your greatest creative potential. When you sleep, your emotional memories are somehow "set" in the brain; this may explain why we tend to function at our best, both mentally and creatively, right after a solid night's sleep.

Primo Athletic Performance: Sleep is one of the most important activities for a successful athlete. I continue to find it amazing how I can go to sleep after a day of strenuous physical activity, feeling bone tired, only to wake up the following morning feeling refreshed. Appropriate sleep does wonders to rejuvenate both mind and body.

Optimum Grades: It stands to reason that if your brain repairs itself while you sleep, you will be able to think clearest in school after a good night of it. Of course, a solid, protein-rich breakfast will help, but the foundation of a productive learning experience remains a healthy chunk of time set aside for sleep.

Managed Stress: Just as sleep helps your body manage and recover from pain, so sleep is essential to managing stress. In our increasingly stressed-out culture, the ability to de-stress is growing in importance. If you are feeling stressed out, taking time out for a nap may help you feel better. Good sleep also allows you to think more clearly in order to resolve whatever is the root cause of your stress.

Chapter 2: How We <u>Don't</u> Sleep

Now you know how much sleep you need and what sleep does for you, but do you know exactly *why* you need to get enough sleep? The consequences of inadequate sleep go far beyond being grouchy the next day. Here are some possible consequences that occur when you don't get enough sleep:

Accidents: A number of vehicle and workplace accidents have been attributed to someone not getting enough sleep. The greatest danger comes from getting seven hours of sleep or less on a regular basis. In the United States, every year approximately 100,000 accidents occur as a result of a driver being too tired. Studies have shown that when you do not get enough sleep, your reaction time can slow as dramatically as if you were legally drunk.

When it comes to the workplace, employees with a history of more than one accident usually also suffer from a lack of sleep. Inadequate sleep contributes to increased sick days, compared to employees who regularly get enough sleep.

Serious Health Issues: When you are not sleeping properly, you are at a much higher risk for potentially fatal health problems, including:

- Heart disease

- Depression

- High blood pressure

- Diabetes

- Heart attack

- Obesity

- Irregular heart beat

- Stroke

Cognitive Difficulties: When it comes to learning and thinking, your brain must be rested and ready to process information. If you are not getting enough sleep, the following are impaired:

- Attention

- Concentration

- Problem solving

- Alertness

- Reasoning

Your memories are consolidated as you sleep. Not getting enough sleep results in difficulty remembering things that you experienced and learned the previous day.

Reduced Sex Drive: If your sex drive is subpar and you have no underlying physical conditions, you might want to look at your sleeping habits. In addition to affecting your libido, lack of sleep can cause you to feel sleepy (as if *that's* a surprise) or lethargic and can actually cause an increase in tension, all of which may work against your sex drive.

Lack of sleep can result in reduced testosterone levels for males. Since this hormone is critical for a man's sex drive, anything that reduces the amount of testosterone can work against normal sexual expression.

Skin Aging: If you want to look as young as possible for as long as possible, you need to make sleep a priority. You really do need your "beauty sleep. " Think about how your skin looks after just a single night of inadequate sleep. You have dark circles under your eyes, you may have puffy eyes or sallow skin. Now, think about how bad these problems can get if your sleep is shortchanged on a regular basis.

Cortisol production is usually suspended during a full night of sleep. When your sleep is interrupted or reduced, your body continues to produce more of this hormone. Excess amounts of cortisol inhibit skin elasticity, as the collagen in your skin starts to break down.

While you suffer from overproduction of cortisone when you don't sleep enough, missing sleep also means your body cannot produce adequate human growth hormone. This hormone is what ensures thick, healthy skin, so a shortage of human growth hormone can cause your skin to become fragile and thin, making your body less capable of repelling attacks to your immune system. A deficit in this hormone can also reduce muscle mass and decrease overall bone strength.

Increased Risk of Anxiety and Depression: If your mood is increasingly grumpy, angry, or sad and if you find you do not care as much about things you normally enjoy, you may be facing the onset of depression. Studies show that people who sleep less than six hours per night are at an increased risk of anxiety and depression.

Depression can also generate insomnia, the inability to get adequate sleep. The two diagnoses often go hand in hand and often feed each other.

Getting enough sleep can help to reduce your depression risk. Of course, getting the right treatment for depression can also help improve your sleep.

Reduced Memory Ability: If you want a strong memory, you need to ensure that you are getting enough sleep. During deep sleep (stages three and four), your brain is storing your long-term memories. If you do not get enough sleep during these sleep stages, you will notice it is harder to recall information and remember events.

Impaired Judgment: You are not able to properly interpret the implications of your choices when you are tired. This includes the inability to accurately assess how your lack of sleep is affecting you! Remember this the next time you tell yourself "Just a few more minutes; I want to finish this page," and a few minutes invariably turn into an hour, all because your judgment (and possibly your sense of time) is impaired.

Impaired judgment can lead to unwise decisions that result in major consequences you have to live with for the rest of your life. Remember that being sleep deprived is almost like being drunk; think about the poor decisions that drunken people tend to make.

Increased Risk of Death: Research shows that sleep deprivation can almost double the risk of death. For example, a sleep-deprived individual with heart disease is almost twice as likely to die as a heart disease patient who gets adequate sleep. The link between sleep deprivation and increased risk of death appears to be most prominent in people with cardiovascular disease.

Weight Gain: Many people who are sleep deprived are at least slightly overweight. When you are not getting enough sleep, you tend to have a greater appetite and feel hungry more often. This is because ghrelin, a peptide known as "the hunger hormone," is more present in sleep deprived people. Another hormone, leptin, which works to suppress the appetite, is reduced by lack of sleep. This can explain why you get the munchies when you are up late at night.

When you are tired, you are more likely to reach for unhealthy foods. Impaired judgment due to sleep deprivation, coupled with an overabundance of ghrelin, can easily influence you to reach for foods that are high in carbohydrates and fat.

Sleep and Body Systems

Lack of sleep affects all systems of your body. It will help to know the symptoms associated with damage to these systems, so you can recognize them should they occur. Here is a brief overview of these symptoms and a little of what can go wrong.

Central Nervous System: Your nervous system is one of the primary body systems affected by lack of sleep. Your nervous system is like a super highway for information, so even the slightest reduction in speed or alteration of normal functioning can yield profound effects across the entire body.

When you are sleeping, your brain's neurons are able to take a rest and at the same time build fresh neural pathways. Your brain also works to repair cell damage caused by the production of proteins necessary for this job.

When your brain is not functioning appropriately due to lack of sleep, the primary symptom – not surprisingly – is sleepiness. People often feel sluggish and say they cannot concentrate. Learning and memory are impacted and people are more prone to experiencing mood swings when the central nervous system is prevented from regenerating itself while you sleep.

If you go without sleep for an extended period of time, you may experience hallucinations, especially if you also have a condition like lupus or narcolepsy. Individuals with bipolar disorder are at a higher risk of experiencing manic episodes. Other possible symptoms that may arise due to the stress on your nervous system include depression, suicidal thoughts, impulsive behavior, and paranoia.

Respiratory System: Respiratory problems, such as influenza and the common cold are more likely in people who are sleep-deprived. It is also possible for lack of sleep to exacerbate existing chronic lung disease.

Immune System: A lack of sleep also weakens your immune system. The immune system produces cells and antibodies that fight infection. These help to fight off viruses, bacteria and other foreign invaders. Cytokines defend your body against illness and energize the entire immune system.

While you are sleeping, your immune system essentially works to strengthen its army. Therefore, if you are short on sleep, your immune system will lack enough soldiers to successfully defend against foreign invaders. The results: you get sick.

Cardiovascular System: Cardiovascular disease is a likely possibility in people who are sleep-deprived. Many of these symptoms stem from the weight gain that can result from lack of sleep.

Your heart and blood vessels also get some necessary repair while you are sleeping. If that repair is interrupted or prevented due to lack of sleep, cardiovascular issues may result. High blood pressure is a common symptom related to lack of sleep. In fact, your blood pressure becomes elevated after a single night of inadequate sleep.

Digestive System: As we have already stated, weight gain is a definite risk when you are sleep deprived. As we discussed earlier, levels of leptin are reduced, resulting in a stronger appetite, while an increase in cortisol levels may lead to excessive fat storage.

Your body also tends to produce greater levels of insulin after you eat. If you eat more, you increase your risk of contracting Type 2 diabetes, which may also increase the amount of fat stored by your body.

Chapter 3: Common Sleep Problems

Everyone has sleeping troubles at some point, but when this becomes a common problem, it is time to talk to your doctor. Sleep issues are common and – if they are ongoing – they can wreak havoc on your overall health. If your sleeping troubles last more than two weeks, it is time to talk to your doctor to see if an underlying physical condition is the cause. A prompt diagnosis can result in treatment to alleviate the root cause as well as reversing any physical imbalances or damage caused by the extended lack of sleep you have experienced.

Insomnia

The most common sleeping problem people experience is insomnia. In most cases, insomnia is a symptom of an underlying cause, be it external events or internal health issues. Insomnia prevents you from falling asleep or from sleeping through the entire night.

A number of causes can trigger insomnia. Some are under your control, but others...not so much. The most common insomnia triggers are:

- Stressful relationships

- Depression or anxiety

- Certain medical conditions

- Certain medications

- Changes in work schedule or environment

- Nicotine, caffeine or alcohol

- Poor sleeping habits

- Eating too close to bedtime

Your doctor can typically diagnose insomnia by learning more about your general health, sleep habits, and your lifestyle. Treatment usually involves addressing the underlying condition and may include medications. Other treatment options work to alter your behavior and can include:

- Sleep hygiene education

- Relaxation techniques

- Sleep restriction

- Light therapy

- Cognitive behavioral therapy

- Stimulus control

- Remaining passively awake

Sleep Apnea

Sleep apnea is not uncommon and it can severely threaten your health. There are two primary types of sleep apnea. Most common is obstructive sleep apnea, which is caused by the relaxation of the throat muscles. The other type – central sleep apnea - occurs when the muscles that control your breathing do not receive appropriate signals from the brain. This condition can manifest in many symptoms, some of which are serious, including:

- Excessive daytime sleepiness

- Sore throat and dry mouth

- Difficulty staying asleep

- Loud snoring

- Morning headaches

- Attention reduction

Obstructive sleep apnea is largely preventable for many people. Knowing the causes can aid in your prevention efforts. The most common sources of obstructive sleep apnea are:

- Excess weight

- Narrowed airway

- Smoking

- Large neck circumference

- Nasal congestion

- Use of sedatives, alcohol or tranquilizers

While central sleep apnea is less common, brain tumors, a stroke and heart disorders are the known causes. If your sleep apnea does not respond to treatment for symptoms of the obstructive type, your doctor may look for causes in terms of central sleep apnea.

The most common method of diagnosing this condition is to take a sleeping test. A sleeping test consists of spending the night in a sleep lab where a healthcare professional monitors your heartbeat, brain activity, lungs and breathing activity, blood oxygen levels, and limb movement as you sleep.

The most common treatment is the CPAP machine because this ensures that you are getting oxygen as you sleep. Other similar devices include the EPAP, adjustable airway pressure devices and certain oral appliances. If these methods fail, your doctor may recommend surgery to ensure a patent airway as you sleep. These procedures may include:

- Tissue removal

- Soft palate implants

- Jaw repositioning

- Creating a new air passage

Restless Leg Syndrome

Restless leg syndrome is a relatively new diagnosis, which can impact your ability to sleep well. When you have this condition, your legs demand to move in order to release tension and pain or to alleviate a vague discomfort. This condition is triggered when you relax, and can both hinder and interrupt sleep, to the point of causing serious sleep deprivation.

While the cause of this condition is unknown, the syndrome tends to be hereditary and there is evidence that it may be linked to low iron levels in the brain. It also is connected to patients with rheumatoid arthritis or diabetes. So far there is no cure for restless legs, but treatments can lessen the symptoms.

A doctor is able to diagnose this condition based upon a physical examination and your report of your symptoms. To identify any contributing causes, your doctor may order blood testing, a neurological examination, or a sleep test.

Medications are commonly used to treat this condition, including:

- Gabapentin

- Anti-convulsants

- Dopamine-decreasing medications, although they sometimes exacerbate the symptoms

- Sleep medications

- Opioid medications

- Muscle relaxers

Narcolepsy

Narcolepsy results from a brain mechanism dysfunction that causes uncontrollable sleepiness during the day. People with this disorder randomly fall asleep, even when they are doing things like driving, talking or working. In addition to excessive sleepiness during the day, other symptoms can include:

- Sleep paralysis

- Sudden muscle tone loss

- Hallucinations

Your doctor will do a number of tests to see if you have this disorder and to see how severe it is. These include:

- **Sleep history:** Your doctor will start with learning more about how you sleep and about how your sleep impacts your wakeful hours. This often includes the Epworth Sleepiness Scale to see how you fare during the day.

- **Polysomnogram:** This test looks at how your heart and brain function during sleep.

- **Hypocretin test:** This is a brain chemical that ensures REM sleep regulation. Your levels of hypocretin are tested by obtaining a sample of spinal fluid.

- **Multiple sleep latency test:** This will help to determine how quickly you fall asleep during daytime hours by having you take several naps, with two hours in between each nap.

Medications are the most common method of treatment. Your doctor may prescribe more than one medicine in order to regulate your sleep cycle and deal with your symptoms. The most common medications include:

- Antidepressants including SNRI medications, tricyclic medications and SSRI medications

- Stimulants

- Sodium oxybate

Jetlag

Jetlag affects your circadian rhythm and makes it hard to sleep and be awake at the proper times. It occurs when you cross time zones and is a temporary issue. Symptoms of jetlag include:

- Disturbed sleep

- Difficulty concentrating

- General malaise

- Daytime fatigue

- Menstrual problems in women

- Muscle soreness

- Gastrointestinal problems

In most cases, treatment is not necessary. However, if you travel often, halcion and certain other sleeping medications can help helpful. Light therapy is another option that helps you regulate your sleep cycle.

Delayed Sleep Phase Syndrome

This condition is characterized by taking at least two hours after one's normal bedtime to fall asleep. If it takes this long to fall asleep, it is only natural that you will find it difficult to rise at the usual time without experiencing some of the symptoms of sleep deprivation. Delayed sleep phase syndrome is most common in among adolescents. Your doctor will explore your symptoms and your sleep habits to make an accurate diagnosis. There are a number of treatments available; most people use a combination of them to sleep easier. Treatments include:

- Improving bedtime habits

- Going to bed slightly earlier each night for several nights, to reset the body's clock

- Using bright light therapy in the morning to reset the internal clock

- Avoiding bright lights before bedtime

- Keeping the bedroom completely dark at night

- Use of sleep medications as prescribed by a doctor

Sleepwalking

Sleepwalking is not an uncommon occurrence in reality. It is considered a type of behavior disorder. Sleepwalking can occur in people of all ages, but shows up most frequently in children aged three to seven. Most sleepwalkers do more than just walk around while they are sleeping. Symptoms can include:

- Walking around

- Difficulty waking a sleepwalker

- Talking while asleep

- Screaming

- Inappropriate behavior

- Little or no memory of sleepwalking

To diagnose this condition, doctors typically perform a sleep study. This gives doctors a clear understanding of what is happening in your body while you are sleeping. If an underlying sleep dysfunction is causing your sleepwalking, treatment typically resolves the issue. Medications and self-hypnosis may also prove beneficial in helping you sleep throughout the night without sleepwalking.

Shift Work Disorder

If you word different shifts at different times, you will likely find it hard to sleep at least some of the time. Once your body gets used to sleeping at a specific time and you switch to another shift, it will take time to adjust to the new sleep schedule. However, there are strategies you can employ to minimize the disruption to your sleep schedule after you change shifts. Even if you are sleeping during the day and working at night, you can know the benefits of a good "night's" sleep.

Use the following tips to help yourself get better sleep even when you are switching shifts periodically:

- If at all possible, try to limit how frequently you have to switch between shifts. This allows your body to better know when it needs to sleep and when it needs to be awake.

- Avoid caffeine toward the end of your shift. You want to be able to sleep after you get off work and caffeine will only keep you awake longer.

- Use lights when you need to wake up and keep it dark when it is time for bed. If you work nights and come home early in the day, wear sunglasses as you make your way home, in order to prevent the sunlight from triggering your body to stay awake.

- On your days off, be sure to get a full night's sleep so your body will remain at top functionality throughout the workweek.

- If you have a long commute that prevents you from getting to sleep quickly after work, consider either finding a job closer to home or arranging with a nearby friend to rent or borrow a bed between workdays.

- During your shift, do what you can to keep yourself moving around and active exerting yourself. This is especially important early in your shift, if you want to sleep well when you go to bed.

- If you have to sleep during the day, you should do everything possible to keep your bedroom quiet and dark. Blackout curtains keep the sunlight out and you can use ear plugs or a white noise machine to minimize noisy distractions. Sometimes just the sound of a fan will be enough to block out external sounds and allow you to sleep peacefully.

Medical Conditions that can Cause Sleep Problems

A number of diseases can also include sleep issues as a symptom. If you have these conditions, you need to know how they affect your sleep so you can take the right steps to maximize your ability to get adequate sleep.

ADHD: You have surely heard of ADHD, but most people see it as more of a daytime problem than something that can cause trouble with sleep. People with this disorder are more likely to feel sleepy during the day. They also have a tendency toward insomnia. Some of the problems may be due to the medications used to treat ADHD, but others are due to the hyperactivity component of the disorder itself.

Asthma: When you have asthma, your lungs can become inflamed, making it difficult to breathe. Some experts believe that asthma can negatively impact your circadian rhythm, making it hard to maintain a normal sleeping cycle. Many asthmatic people also have trouble sleeping because of wheezing, coughing and feeling breathless at night. Symptoms can make it difficult to fall asleep; they can also interrupt sleep to the point that sleep deprivation becomes an additional issue to contend with.

Alzheimer's Disease: This disease can negatively affect your circadian rhythm, resulting in the inability to sleep on a normal schedule. People with Alzheimer's tend to fall asleep during the day and wake during odd hours of the night. How severely their sleep is impacted generally depends upon the severity of the disease. The more severe the Alzheimer's symptoms, the worse the sleeping issues become.

COPD: Chronic obstructive pulmonary disease makes it hard to breathe. Chest pain, coughing and frequent urination all are part of this condition and each can wreak havoc on a person's sleep. Sleep problems may also result from some of the medications that people use to treat COPD. Some of the inhalers contain steroids, which can you up at night because of their stimulating effect.

Depression: Sleep issues are one of the most common problems that occur during depression. Some people find they are sleeping far too much because they don't want to wake in the morning. Others are unable to sleep at all due to a racing brain that refuses to stop bouncing off the walls. Both issues contribute to excessive sleepiness during the day and other symptoms of sleep deprivation.

Dementia: Dementia patients often experience disturbed sleep and may wander during the night. Tranquilizers tend to worsen the symptoms, leaving the person confused upon waking. Other medications are available, but these tend to have bad side effects and may actually make the sleeping issues even worse.

GERD: Gastroesophageal Reflux Disease, commonly associated with acid reflux and heartburn, can cause pain and burning in your chest and stomach which interferes with sleep. People who have this condition are also more likely to develop other health problems that can interrupt sleep, such as sleep apnea, insomnia, and restless leg syndrome. The lack of sleep contributes to being foggy and sleepy during the day, symptoms, once again, associated with sleep deprivation.

Epilepsy: Epilepsy is a condition where you experience seizures that can range from brief moments of unawareness to full blown grand mal seizures in which the body moves erratically, outside the control of the individual. Due to the effects that epilepsy has on the brain, experts often associate it with sleeping difficulties. In fact, it is possible to experience seizures while you are sleeping. Epileptic seizures, whenever they are experienced, can result in concentration problems and intense fatigue during the day.

Multiple Sclerosis: This is an autoimmune condition that affects the nerves. Difficulty sleeping is one of the most common symptoms among people who have this condition. Then, when you are fatigued under MS, this can exacerbate other symptoms, such as balance issues, muscle pain, spasticity, and memory. The sleep issues are generally associated with not getting a restful sleep due to waking up frequently throughout the night.

Fibromyalgia: This condition is most known for causing pain throughout the body, but many people also experience sleep disturbances. Those with this condition are typically fatigued as a symptom with the inability to sleep well further contributing to a person's fatigue. Not getting enough sleep can also worsen other symptoms of this condition, such as mental fogginess and muscle pain.

Allergies: When you have allergies, your stuffed-up sinuses can make it difficult to breathe through your nose. An itchy nose and frequent sneezing can also interrupt an otherwise peaceful night. Many people with allergies find they sleep poorly during particularly bad episodes. Due to the lack of sleep, they will feel tired during the day and find it extremely difficult to concentrate on everyday tasks. Allergies can also cause you to wake up with a sore throat or a dry mouth, further disrupting sleep and sometimes preventing the sufferer from easily falling back to sleep.

Pain: When you are in pain, it is hard to get comfortable and if you cannot get comfortable, you cannot sleep. This is a common problem; even those with minor aches and pains may find that their sleep is disturbed. This can be a vicious cycle because when you are not getting enough rest, it is common to experience a worsening of your pain. It is important to work on both issues simultaneously to find a positive resolution to your suffering.

When it comes to medical conditions that cause sleep deprivation, your doctor will usually inquire about how it is affecting your sleep. If your medical professional does not ask, do initiate the discussion. Sleep deprivation is important to address, because sometimes either the treatment for the condition is causing your sleeping troubles your condition may not being treated adequately in order to allow you to sleep. Sleep deprivation, while usually temporary, can seriously impact your body's ability to heal itself. In light of this, it would behoove you to persist in working with the medical staff to fix your sleeping problems so that you can finally get some rest.

There are some cases where your doctor will add to your treatment regimen to help keep your condition under control. This may include sleeping medications. However, if your condition only affects your sleep some of the time, your doctor may recommend an over-the-counter medication or supplement to help you sleep on those occasions.

Chapter 4: Energize Your Morning

Even after a good night's sleep, you may wake up feeling tired and unrefreshed. This is normally the time when people start reaching for the caffeine. However, you already know caffeine can cause jitteriness without actually improving your situation. In this instance, you will want to find alternative ways to get that morning boost of energy. The good news is that you can easily feel awake and alert in the morning within minutes of waking, when you use the right tips and techniques.

Move Around: As soon as you roll over and turn off your alarm, immediately get out of bed and start moving around. This increases your blood pressure and heart rate, helping you feel more awake and alert. Within about ten minutes, you will find you are feeling more awake and that your energy levels are increasing. If you need to, can even take a short walk around the block, especially in the warmer months when you can get the most sunshine.

Choose the Right Breakfast: What you choose to eat in the morning impacts the rest of your day. You want to eat foods that gently increase your blood sugar. Sugary breakfasts may jolt your body into high alert status, but after the sugar spike is over, your glucose levels will crash and you'll find yourself tired and hungry, well before time for a break.

A mixture of complex carbohydrates and protein are always ideal. This wakes up your digestive system and gives you energy that will sustain you across the next several hours. An excellent starter would be some organic peanut butter on whole wheat or twelve-grain toast.

Yogurt is always a good option, especially if you toss in some fresh fruit and nuts. Oatmeal is also a good choice, due to its healthy carbohydrates; just add a few pieces of turkey sausage or bacon for a blast of protein. These foods provide a boost of energy that can keep you going until lunch time.

Make it Bright: Open up your curtains to let the sunshine in or turn on some lights. Bright light helps to increase your alertness and reduce sleepiness. You can do this as you are taking ten minutes to walk around your house in the morning. If your home or apartment does not provide a lot of sunlight, consider taking five minutes to just stand or walk outside in the sun. Light will help your body know it is time to be awake.

One useful tool to help you wake, especially if you live in a place where the days are short in winter, is an alarm clock that gradually brightens your room starting thirty minutes before the alarm goes off. These sunrise clocks actually simulate a natural sunrise.

Talk to Someone: A conversation first thing in the morning can also help you wake up. It stimulates you to use your mind, which gently nudges your brain to gear up for the day. You do not have to seek out deep and meaningful conversation; just talk to the people who are up and about as you are getting ready in the morning. The key is to ensure that the conversation is positive and keeps you alert and actively thinking for at least fifteen minutes.

Drink Some Water: Start your morning off with a tall glass of ice cold water. This naturally perks you up so you can take on the day. Don't chug it down all at once, but sip on your water as you go about your morning routine.

Get Some Exercise: People who engage in morning exercise often report that it almost immediately wakes them up. They also often state that it gives them more energy throughout the day. In the morning hours, you want to increase your heart rate and blood pressure, so a morning cardio session is the best option. An outside walk can also be stimulating to the whole body and refreshing to the soul. If you exercise regularly during the day, you will also find that it is a lot easier to fall asleep at night.

Ignore Work and School: When you first wake up in the morning, it is easy for your mind to automatically start zeroing in on the things you need to do throughout the day. However, it is best to focus on things that do not cause stress first thing in the morning. Stress can make you tired, working against your desire to be alert when you first get started with your day. Steer your thoughts toward things that make you happy or fun things you are looking forward to. Granted, this will be easier if you have planned and prepared for your day back before you went to bed yesterday, but we will discuss pre-bedtime routines in further detail later in the book.

Sing a Song: Singing is a great way to boost your morning energy because it can stimulate body, mind, and spirit, sometimes providing a true emotional high. It also increases a positive outlook and decreases stress. When you are getting ready in the morning, put on some tunes you love and start singing along. When you get in the car to head to work or school, bring an energizing song mix with you so you can carry the joy with you as you go. By the time you reach your destination, you will be alert and better equipped to face whatever the day throws at you.

Smell Some Cinnamon: The scent of cinnamon works to reduce fatigue, making it the perfect morning scent. Keep cinnamon sticks in your dressing area or light a cinnamon-scented candle to set the mood for an energetic and productive day ahead. If you are not a cinnamon fan, grab some peppermint. Smell it or pop a peppermint into your mouth as you are getting ready; this can also increase your energy.

Watch Something Funny: Remember how you used to watch cartoons as a kid while you were getting ready in the morning? Feel free to reintroduce this habit into your life for a morning energy boost. Find a comical show and have a few laughs while you are getting dressed and coiffed.

Open Your Eyes to Beauty: When you awake in the morning, you want the first thing you to your eyes to be something that makes you happy. Put a picture of your favorite people next to your alarm. You can also put a vase of fresh flowers in that area so that you see flowers right away and you get the bonus of the scent of fresh flowers in your bedroom.

Take a Power Shower: Choose shower products that have an energizing scent. Go for clean and citrusy smells, which are known to be invigorating. Use warm and not hot water, since hot water can be a little too relaxing when you're winding up for the day. You also want to keep your bathroom as bright as possible to reinforce your body clock. If you can pump some natural sunlight into the room, that's all the better.

Get Some Orange Juice: Fresh squeezed orange juice is known to be energizing and it is the perfect breakfast beverage. You can combine it with any breakfast that you choose. Simply make some fresh orange juice the night before so that it is ready to go when you are preparing to have your breakfast in the morning. You can also take a cup of it on the go to drink as you complete your commute to work.

Chapter 5: Best Daytime Habits

How you spend your day has a major impact on how well you are able to sleep at night. You will be amazed how a few tweaks to your daytime schedule can contribute to an increased ability to sleep peacefully when you go to bed. In this chapter you will be able to affirm your existing good habits and likely add a few new ones that will position you to get the best sleep available at the end of your day. You will also learn how each habit contributes to healthy sleep as well as productive waking time.

Complete Your To-Do List Early: This is very important because you do not want to run around your home trying to get things finished right before you go to bed. Such activity only stimulates mind and body, making it harder to unwind and relax when you do stop running and lie down. I advise reworking your schedule so that everything you need to accomplish is completed at least by three hours before bedtime. This gives you a few hours of unwind time so that you can prepare your mind and body for sleep.

Prepare for the Next Day: At the end of your workday, you should take stock of what you have accomplished and briefly plan your activities for the following day. When you are at home, I suggest preparing your next day's lunch and snacks so all you have to do is grab them when you are ready to go. Also, to save your mind from the stress of half-awake decision-making, I recommend you select your clothes for the next day and set them out so they will be easy to access in the morning.

Watch the Caffeine Consumption: Drinking a cup of coffee in the morning is fine and usually will not interfere with your sleep that night. However, if you are still consuming caffeine into the evening hours, your body is going to remain stimulated. About eight hours before your bedtime, stop consuming anything that contains caffeine. You also want to limit your caffeine consumption throughout the day to avoid over-stimulation at any point.

Turn Off Electronics Early: Today, it is common for people to bring electronics to bed with them, but this can make it harder to get to sleep. About thirty minutes before you head to bed, you want to power everything off and focus on your pre-bed routine. This means no television, computers, phones or anything else that can leave you stimulated. You want to focus only on relaxing routines and activities at this time, to prime yourself for a good night of sleep.

Nap Wisely: A quick nap can be a good way to recharge yourself during the day, but if your naps are too long or too late in the day, they can interfere with your sleep. If you need a nap, keep it to no longer than thirty minutes. You also want to avoid napping at least six hours before you normally go to bed. It is best to use other energizing techniques and avoid naps completely, especially if you are prone to experiencing insomnia.

Exercise Early: Exercise does a lot to help you sleep well, but schedule your exercise toward the early part of the day. This helps provide energy that lasts throughout the day and also aids in preparing your body for sleep at night. You should include a good mixture of strength training and cardiovascular exercises in order to promote health and optimum sleep. Ideally, you will want to exercise in the morning or afternoon for the best sleep-inducing benefits.

Eat Magnesium: This mineral helps you sleep better, so eating it with your dinner is a good option for promoting sleep at night. You can add some leafy green vegetables, black beans, or pumpkin seeds to your dinner to get a good dose of magnesium. If you are deficient in this nutrient, talk to your doctor about taking a high-quality supplement. The main priority is getting an appropriate daily intake of magnesium, in order to experience healthy sleep.

Sugar Warning: If you eat sugar too late in the day, you will spike your insulin levels making it harder to fall asleep. As much as possible, avoid ingesting sugar following your lunch hour so that you can start preparing your body for nighttime sleep. Avoiding sugar allows your body to recover from any insulin spikes that have occurred in the day, so that you are not left lying awake for a long period of time at night.

Hop Out of Bed: People who hit the snooze button in the morning often find it harder to fall asleep at night. When your alarm sounds, make it a point to get right out of bed and start your morning routine. This helps to increase your alertness and give your body the message that it is time to kick into gear and start functioning. You may think there is so much time between waking and heading to bed that it makes no difference, but trust me; if you get going first thing in the morning, you are helping to improve your nighttime sleep quality.

Maintain a Daily Journal: After you enjoy dinner, take ten to fifteen minutes to write in your journal. Research shows that people who take the time to write about the positive aspects of their day at around this time are able to sleep better at night. Journaling will also allow you to vent any negative thoughts or energy, so that they will not weigh on your mind, keeping you agitated at bedtime.

Standard Wakeup Time: You should awake at the same time seven days a week. This is very important. If you keep a regular sleeping schedule, your body will become used to sleeping during those specific hours. After a while, your body will start automatically preparing for sleep, making it much more likely that you can fall asleep and get adequate rest each night.

Spend Time Outdoors: People who spend a lot of time outdoors tend to sleep better at night. This is because absorbing sunlight during the day helps to regulate your circadian rhythm, also known as your body clock. Your body interprets daylight as the time to be awake and active. It will also sense, once it starts to get dark, that it is time to start producing melatonin in preparation for falling asleep at night. The more consistently you live within these daily boundaries, the easier it will be to get the sleep you need.

Chapter 6: Your Bedtime Routine

Having a solid sleeping routine is a proven way to improve how well you can sleep at night. There are many things you can incorporate into your routine in order to reap the maximum benefits from the sleep time that follows. Many people just go to bed at night and do not allow their mind and body to prepare for sleep. This can lead to insomnia or frequent awakening as you try to settle into sleep. A great routine can mean productive sleep and a more energetic tomorrow.

Establish a Sleep Schedule

This is the first step in creating your nighttime routine because you need to start preparing your body. If your body knows when it is time for bed, it will be easier to sleep well. Set a regular bedtime and make sure that you stick to this every night of the week. This is critical and it has been proven to help reduce insomnia. You can start tonight by selecting a specific bedtime and going to bed at the time you set.

If you normally go to bed very late and need to start sleeping several hours earlier, you will need to make this a gradual change in order to prevent insomnia. Each day, head to bed fifteen minutes earlier, until you reach your desired bedtime. This allows you to gently ease your body into sleep.

Boost Melatonin Production

Melatonin is a hormone that helps regulate your sleep-wake cycle. You need to ensure that your body is producing enough at the right time so that you can get a good night's sleep. Use the following tips to encourage your pineal gland to release enough melatonin at the right time:

- About thirty minutes before you go to bed, turn off all electronic devices to reduce stimulation to the mind and body.

- If you read before bed, use an actual book and never a tablet or digital reading device, such as a Nook.

- Swap the light bulbs in your sleeping area for bulbs of a lower wattage. This helps your body avoid misinterpreting the bright lights as sunlight.

- Ensure the bedroom is fully dark. You can fairly easily find curtains that block out the light from streetlamps and the moon. You should also shut all doors in your bedroom so that light does not filter in.

- If you awake in the night for a bathroom break, never turn on the lights. Instead, use a flashlight so the lights do not trick your body into thinking it is daytime.

Optimize Your Sleeping Quarters

Outside of light, the two greatest factors that can interfere with your sleep are noise and an uncomfortable bed. Reduce all noise to avoid being awakened by it during the night. Noise also impacts falling asleep; it tends to focus your mind on what you are hearing, engaging your mind instead of letting it disengage to fall asleep. A comfortable bed ensures that you can fully relax. You might need to switch out your mattress or add a topper if your current bed is not comfortable.

You also will want to regulate the temperature in your room. If the room is too cold or hot, that fact can occupy your mind instead of getting comfortably relaxed. It is best to keep your room a little on the cool side. Do not pile on too many blankets, because you may get too hot and find yourself waking up to remove some of the covers. Select sleep clothes made of a breathable fabric, so that your clothing will not trap your body heat and cause sweat or discomfort from being too warm.

The Four-Hour Warning

Approximately four hours before your scheduled bedtime, you should start preparing for sleep. This is the time to start ramping down your stimulation level to make it easier to get to sleep. At the same time, avoid things that increase your risk of waking up during the night. Here are four main things to focus on that can help you rest easy at night:

- **Avoid Heavy Meals:** If you tend to eat larger dinners, eat early, before this four-hour window begins. Heavy meals sit in your stomach and can cause heartburn, making you too uncomfortable to sleep. They can also keep you awake while your body is trying to digest them.

- **Stop Drinking Alcohol:** Even a single drink within four hours of bedtime can make it harder for you to sleep at night. Alcohol is difficult for your body to metabolize and also has diuretic effects. Avoiding alcohol close to bedtime will minimize the chance of a middle-of-the-night urge to get up and urinate.

- **Reduce Water Intake:** The same holds true for water. Water is great and you need to keep hydrated, but you'll want to restrict water intake four hours before bedtime. Once again, you do not need multiple bathroom trips interrupting your sleep.

- **Do Not Smoke:** Since nicotine is a stimulant, if you are smoking cigarettes close to bedtime, you are keeping your body artificially revved up. Even after you manage to fall asleep, nicotine can prevent you from receiving the restorative benefits of a restful sleep.

Components of a 30-Minute Pre-Bed Ritual

There are a few things you can do thirty minutes before bed that will help you relax. These are activities you can pursue every night until they have become a nightly habit. Your body will get used to these activities and take them as a cue that it is time for bed. You can choose two or three of the following to help yourself get better sleep:

- Take a warm, leisurely bath to relax your body and relieve the effects of stress.

- Drink a caffeine-free herbal tea, such as valerian, lavender or chamomile; each of these help relaxation and promote sleep.

- Have a small snack that includes sleep-inducing foods (discussed later in this book).

- Perform one or two relaxing yoga poses. Check out the YouTube video at https://www.doyogawithme.com/content/yoga-nidra-sleep.

- Spend five minutes meditating to expel negative thoughts and stress.

- Spend a few minutes praying to ease your mind and refresh your spirit. For a helpful example of prayer, see Marce Corona's YouTube entitled "Bedtime Prayer - Sleep knowing that God is taking care of you."

- Read a paperback or hardcover book that is not overly stimulating (something that proceeds at a relaxed pace and is soothing to the emotions).

- Play white noise.

- Dim the lights.

Avoid all work, schoolwork and other activities that require concentration during the thirty minutes before bedtime. This is your time to decompress and get your body ready for sleep. Set apart this time for things that are relaxing and help you let go of the stress that has built up over the day. If you need more than thirty minutes, you can alter your routine as required to accommodate. The key is to create a routine that works for you on a regular basis.

How to Get Back to Sleep

Sometimes you wake up and have a hard time getting back to sleep. At those times you can have a brief routine prepared to encourage your body to return to your slumber. Here are a few tips that can keep middle-of-the-night wakeups from depriving you of sleep:

- Take a few minutes to meditate while lying down. I suggest listening to a YouTube video by Doug Hoseck entitled "Guided Meditation Sleep: Go to sleep in 10 minutes." Meditation helps to push any disruptive thoughts out of your mind and ease your return to sleep.

- Read a non-stimulating book for about fifteen minutes to help relax your mind and encourage sleepiness.

- Use visualization to imagine yourself in a comfortable and peaceful place. This can help your body relax and encourage your mind to drift back off to sleep.

Chapter 7: Build A Sleep Sanctuary

You know sleep is critical and where you sleep is one of the most important aspects of getting healthy, rejuvenating sleep. Your bedroom should be a place of tranquility that you only use for sleeping and sex. It is critical that you never use this room for work or anything else; otherwise or your associations with the bedroom may prevent you from fully relaxing and getting proper rest. You need a sanctuary that allows you to relax and sleep peacefully. Here are a few things you can do to turn your bedroom into a sleep sanctuary.

De-Clutter the Bedroom

If your bedroom is full of clutter, it will not give off the tranquil vibe you need. Dedicate one of your days off to removing all of the clutter from your bedroom. Keep decorative pieces to a minimum and remove piles. You want a clean and minimal space, since clutter can cause stress and stress makes it harder to sleep. All you really need in your room are a few decorative pieces, a bed, a bedside table, a dresser, and a chair.

Choose the Best Bed and Bedding

Your bed is your most important piece of bedroom furniture. It must provide maximum comfort, or else you will not rest well. Two of the most popular mattress types are memory foam and air mattresses. Both have their benefits and allow you to sleep comfortably. Compared to a box-spring mattress, these beds will always be more comfortable and will allow you to sink into the mattress while ensuring that your bones and joints are aligned properly.

You can use the following questions to help you to evaluate if you need a new mattress:

- When you awake in the morning, are you in pain?

- Does your mattress have visible wear and tear?

- Is your mattress at least seven years old?

- Do you sleep better elsewhere?

When it comes to bedding, you want to focus on sheets and blankets that are comfortable and help you to maintain a stable body temperature. It is always best to use fabrics that allow air to circulate freely, such as cotton. With breathable fabrics, you will keep cool and the chances are much lower of overheating in your sleep and waking up to cool off.

Choose a pillow that is able to properly support your neck in your preferred sleeping position. This will prevent you from waking up with a strained and sore neck. I recommend seeking advice from your chiropractor or orthopedist as to the best pillow for your body. You should test out pillows to see that they conform properly to your neck's natural curve. You should also promptly replace your pillows once they start to wear down; you want to prevent them from becoming too flat to properly support your head.

Remove Area Rugs and Regularly Clean Curtains and Bedding

It is important that the things in your room are not able to hold onto allergens. This is especially important if you have allergies or a condition that affects your breathing. If your nose gets stuffy at night, not only may you find it difficult to stay asleep, but the extra effort it takes to breathe and the subsequent reduction in oxygen to your body may reduce its ability to fully regenerate at night. Keeping allergens out of your room is fairly simple. You can maintain a healthy bedroom by following these tips:

- Use curtains that are washable and easy to clean. About once a month, take down your curtains and wash them to minimize dust accumulation.

- Swap out your bedding for fresh linens at least once a week

- Avoid putting area rugs in your room, since they can trap allergens and be troublesome to keep clean

- Dust all surfaces weekly, using a moist cloth or a dust-trapping duster

- Clean your bedroom floor each week to pick up and remove any dust that has accumulated

- If your room has a fan, clean all surfaces at least once a month

Control the Temperature

If you can control the temperature in your room, you will find it easier to sleep. A temperature of approximately sixty-five degrees Fahrenheit is ideal for a sleeping sanctuary. If you cannot control your bedroom temperature separately, I suggest turning the temperature of the entire house to this temperature, just at night. You can also use a very quiet fan if you tend to get warm in your sleep.

Pick the Right Lighting

You need the lighting in your bedroom to be relaxing and ambient. Avoid using bright light bulbs at night; keep your lights between forty-five and sixty watts. This ensures that you have enough light to get around safely, but it is not so bright that your body will think it is daytime. You should have a maximum of two lamps in your room with lightbulbs of this wattage. Avoid using overhead lights at night because they tend to be too bright.

Pick the Right Colors

Color can have a major impact on your mood and your ability to relax. Stick to low-key earth tones in your bedroom to help you feel relaxed and comfortable. Avoid bright red, pink, orange, and yellow. These colors are stimulating and can keep you awake even when your room is dark at night. Employ these calming colors throughout your bedroom, including the walls, the furniture, and all of your bedding.

Choose a Calming Scent

Many people like to release fragrant scents in their bedrooms to provide an overall ambiance of peace. However, energizing scents such as citrus fruits can actually stimulate and keep you awake. Instead, release scents like lavender and chamomile; these are known to be relaxing. You can use essential oils or even fresh herbs to achieve this. Just make sure to keep the scent fresh so that you get the most benefit from it.

Bed Positioning

Avoid placing your bed right under a window or right next to a door if possible. You want to minimize the risk of exposure to light and sounds while you sleep. Choose the darkest and quietest part of your room for your bed. You also want to avoid placing the foot of your bed before a window; otherwise, you risk the uncomfortable wakeup call of the sun shining directly on your face before you're ready to wake up. Keep the windows to one side of your bed and sleep with your back towards them.

Design for Your Personality

While the overall functionality of your sleep sanctuary is the most important, it is also essential that you are happy with how your room looks. Your bedroom should reflect your personality while incorporating the appropriate tips provided in this chapter. When you are changing your bedroom, do take time to think about what you like. Do you have a favorite design style, such as rustic, shabby chic or modern, or are your tastes more of an eclectic mix?

Once you have redesigned, cleaned, and reordered your new sleep sanctuary, take time to rest from your labors, enjoying what you have accomplished. When you love your bedroom and it is designed appropriately for your needs and tastes, you may notice that you sleep more peacefully at night.

Chapter 8: Sleep Hygiene and Natural Remedies

Sleep hygiene is one of the most important aspects of getting appropriate sleep at night. Sleep includes the rituals and habits that you use to improve your ability to sleep. Thankfully, you can do a number of things to improve your sleep hygiene to ensure that you are getting the right amount of restful sleep every night. Explore these tips and start working them into your sleep hygiene practices today, in order to improve your sleep:

- Make sure that you wake up and head to bed at the same time each day. This helps your body to develop a proper circadian rhythm so that you are less likely to fall asleep during the day or experience insomnia in the evenings.

- Make sure that your sleep sanctuary is comfortable and relaxing.

- Your bedroom should only be for sex and sleep. Remove all other distractions and items that can keep you up at night, such as televisions and computers.

- Do not use stimulants, such as nicotine or caffeine, before you go to bed. Even if you fall asleep quickly, these increase the risk of waking in the night.

- Avoid alcohol, because it will make you drowsy and is counterproductive to a deep and restorative sleep. If you have a drink in the evening, it should be at least three to four hours before bed so that it has time to metabolize before you go to bed.

- Never eat anything big or spicy before bed. If your body needs to digest a full meal before you go to bed, you will not get a restful sleep. When it comes to spicy food, this can cause heartburn and make it hard to get comfortable for sleep.

- Make sure to exercise, but not close to bedtime, because it can leave you feeling awake and energized.

- About two hours before you head to bed, you want to minimize your fluid intake. This will reduce the need to get up and go to the bathroom during the night.

- Go to bed when tired. If you are not tired and try to sleep, you will just lie there. Instead, try to do something relaxing to help yourself prepare for a restful night's sleep.

Natural Remedies That Promote Sleep

When it comes to getting more sleep, many people turn to natural remedies so that they can work toward better sleep with a reduced risk of side effects. There are many options and a variety of alternative methods you can explore. It is important to learn more about the remedies so that you can narrow down the best choices for your needs. Before you employ any natural remedies, talk to your doctor to ensure safety and proper use.

Herbs

There are herbs for almost everything and sleep is no exception. Since there are so many herbs that are relaxing and able to promote sleep, it is important to learn more about each one, so you can ensure the best choice for your needs. You can usually take more than one herb at a time, but consult a doctor before mixing herbs or other substances to ensure safety. You should also get help with the proper dosing.

Wild Lettuce: This is an herb you do not hear a lot about, but it has a number of uses that can aid in your quest to improve your sleep. Wild lettuce helps to reduce your anxiety and promotes calmness that can help you sleep even when stressed. It can also help to calm restless leg symptoms, headaches, and pain in your joints or muscles. You should use this particular supplement about thirty minutes before heading to bed to ensure proper rest.

Hops: When you think about hops, you are likely thinking about beer, but hops have many uses that promote sleep. This herb is very calming because it has a mild sedative effect. Some people report that using hops as a sleep remedy actually works at least as well as over-the-counter sleeping medications. About thirty minutes before you go to bed you should take your dose of hops to help you relax and fall asleep.

Valerian: This herb is very commonly used for promoting better sleep. It helps you to fall asleep faster and it improves the overall quality of sleep. Most people receive the most benefit from valerian when they use it over the long-term. This means regular use helps to promote better sleep. There are times when this herb has the opposite effect and promotes energy, but if this happens, taking it during the day can help to promote sleep at night.

Chamomile: Chamomile is known to be a very relaxing herb. It has a sedative effect and is used throughout the world as a remedy for insomnia. Some people drink it as a tea about an hour before bed to relax them and help promote sleep.

Passion Flower: This herb is popular for women's health, but its ability to calm the mind makes it an effective option for sleep, too. It has a sedative effect and is best for insomnia that is not severe, since its sedative effects are rather subtle.

Lavender: The lavender plant works to calm the nervous system. You can use it in capsule form or drink it as tea. To make the tea, simply steep the fresh herb. Drink lavender tea about half an hour before sleep.

California Poppy: This plant is popular throughout the country and research shows that it is effective for reducing anxiety. The poppy has sedative elements that can improve the quality of your sleep, as well as reducing the amount of time it takes to fall asleep. The tea form is the most popular way to ingest this herb.

St. John's Wort: This herb is very popular for improving the mood, but it also contains sleep-promoting properties. It may help to reduce insomnia associated with certain brain chemistry issues.

Kava Kava: This is Fiji's national drink, a potion that helps to calm and relax the body. When individuals find it hard to get to sleep they often use this herb, usually in tea form, for its sedative effects. Kava kava helps you fall asleep and sleep through the night.

Magnolia Bark: This is a sedative that makes you drowsy quickly, so you should not use this herb until you are in bed to ensure safety. It helps to promote sleep by lowering cortisol levels and relaxing your mind.

Ashwagandha: This is a stress-busting herb. While it does not have sedative effects, ashwagandha does help to control anxiety and reduce cortisol so that you are not kept awake by stress, anxiety, or high cortisol levels.

Melatonin

Melatonin is probably one of the most popular natural remedy for promoting sleep. Melatonin is a hormone that is produced by your pineal gland, so some is already in your body. This gland remains inactive during the day. It is activated by darkness; once the sun goes down, it starts to produce melatonin. Blood levels of this hormone increase sharply and remain at a high level for approximately twelve hours.

Some people take a melatonin supplement to increase their melatonin levels and help them to fall asleep faster. It is very important that you take the proper dose of this hormone. I recommend discussing your use of this – and all other supplements – with your healthcare professional. When you take a melatonin supplement it will add to the melatonin already in your body, so proper dosage is vital to your health.

Melatonin can also be a good option for people with jet lag; research suggests that it helps to reset your internal clock. Combining a high-quality melatonin supplement with light therapy can help you establish a proper sleep-wake cycle more quickly. This is a good option for travelers who do not want to miss out on vacation opportunities due to problems with their sleep schedule.

Aromatherapy

The use of aromatherapy goes back for thousands of years. This method uses essential oils to help heal the body and mind. Various scents work for different ailments and several are ideal for helping to promote sleep. Review the oils that are listed below and pick the ones that best work to address your sleeping needs.

When you are using aromatherapy, it is important to properly dilute the oils. The dilution instructions will be on the bottle and dilution ratios will differ from oil to oil. You will dilute your essential oils into a carrier oil, such as jojoba oil. I also highly recommend using an aromatherapy essential oil diffuser that will diffuse a steady fragrance while you sleep.

Chamomile Oil: This oil can be used in a pre-bedtime bath to relax your muscles and help you to sleep. Chamomile calms the body and mind, ensuring a restful night's sleep.

Lavender Oil: Lavender is versatile. It has excellent relaxing properties and helps you to prepare for sleep. It also works as a nervous system tonic to calm frazzled nerves so that they do not cause insomnia.

Vetiver: This oil helps your brain relax and shut down for sleep. You can mix it with lavender to tone down the earthy scent and better induce sleep.

Ylang Ylang: This oil is very relaxing. Simply sniffing this oil before you go to bed helps your body prepare for sleep.

Bergamot: This is a citrus oil, but unlike other citrusy oils, it does not stimulate. It is very calming, allowing you to overcome insomnia.

Nutritional Supplements

There are certain nutritional supplements that are helpful for promoting sleep. You will take these nutrients about an hour before you go to bed to reap the greatest benefits. You should not take sleeping medications or herbs along with these supplements unless your doctor tells you otherwise. You also want to be careful about the dose, because it is possible to overdose on nutritional supplements. Talk to your doctor first to get the right dose and to ensure you are using them safely.

Calcium and Magnesium: Calcium and magnesium both have a similar effect on the body; they work to boost your ability to sleep well during the night. You should take these supplements together when using them to promote sleep.

L-theanine: This is a type of amino acid that works in two ways: it helps to ensure that you sleep deeply at night and it keeps you alert during the day. It is important that you are using a high-quality brand when it comes to this supplement. Poor quality versions may actually block theanine and cause other problems.

Lycopene: This nutrient is getting a lot of attention for its health-promoting benefits. One of the primary benefits is its ability to help regulate your sleep patterns so that you can sleep properly each night.

Selenium: Selenium works similar to lycopene in that it helps to regulate sleep patterns. If you are already working to create a sleep schedule, this supplement can help you to get to sleep at the right time.

What you choose to snack on before bed has a major impact on the quality of your sleep. There are foods that can actually promote sleep and others that can make it harder to sleep. The foods you want to eat in small portions about an hour before bed include:

- **Cherries:** These help control your circadian rhythm for a healthy sleep pattern.

- **Milk:** The old wives' tale that warm milk helps you sleep is an accurate one. Milk promotes sleep because it contains calcium as well as tryptophan, an amino acid that can induce sleep.

- **Bananas:** Bananas are rich in magnesium, a nutrient known for promoting sleep.

- **Turkey:** When you get sleepy after eating holiday dinners, you can thank the turkey. Turkey meat is another food that contains tryptophan, an amino acid that helps you fall asleep.

- **Sweet potato:** Sweet potatoes contain potassium, a nutrient that helps to relax the muscles. This ensures comfort so that you can doze off smoothly.

- **Walnuts:** Walnuts contain melatonin, a hormone that aids in sleep.

- **Almonds:** This nut has a high magnesium content. Magnesium helps to promote sleep.

- **Cheese:** A wedge of cheese can help you sleep because it contains calcium, a sleep-friendly nutrient.

- **Lettuce:** Lettuce contains a compound called lactucarium. This compound provides sedative effects that work almost like opium on the brain.

- **Tuna:** Tuna contains a high level of vitamin B6. This vitamin aids in the production of melatonin.

- **Kale:** Kale is a food rich in calcium. It also contains nutrients that aid the brain in utilizing sleep-inducing tryptophan.

There are also foods you should avoid in order to ensure a restful sleep. Stay away from these foods, starting several hours before you go to bed:

- **Burgers:** Burgers take a lot of time and energy to digest and they can cause heartburn, both of which interfere with sleep.

- **Wine:** That glass of wine might make you drowsy, but drinking it before bed can keep you awake while your body metabolizes it.

- **Coffee:** Coffee works as a stimulant due to its caffeine.

- **Dark chocolate:** Just like coffee, dark chocolate is rich in caffeine which can keep you awake.

- **Soda:** Sodas can contain caffeine, stimulating to your body. Sodas may also increase your need to urinate, waking you up at night to use the bathroom.

- **Spicy foods:** These foods can keep you awake if they cause heartburn.

- **Chicken:** Chicken is typically a healthy food, but it contains a lot of protein which takes a while to digest. The digestion process may keep you awake for a while.

Relaxation Techniques

Relaxation techniques come with a lot of benefits that help you sleep more peacefully. You can combine these with any other sleep treatment or remedy, which makes them highly versatile. The benefits of relaxation techniques include:

- Slowing your heart rate

- Slowing the breathing rate

- Reduction of stress hormone activity

- Reduction in blood pressure

- Decrease in chronic pain

- Decrease in muscle tension

Deep Breathing: This is a technique where you take five to ten deep breaths to clear your mind. Hold each breath for about fifteen seconds and then exhale slowly. You can do this in a warm bath or simply when you are relaxing in bed and preparing to go to sleep.

Massage: Muscle tension and pain can interrupt your sleep. A massage reduces pain and works out tight muscles, allowing your body to relax. Something as simple as a loved one massaging your shoulders for five to ten minutes is enough to help you relax and fall asleep easier. Receiving regular massages from a professional is an even better option if this is something you are able to do.

Meditation: A quiet and peaceful place, such as your bedroom, is essential for meditation. Spend ten minutes fully clearing your mind and imagining your muscles relaxing. Once you finish meditating, you will be better prepared for sleep.

Yoga: You can choose the yoga poses that make you feel the most relaxed and in control. I recommend choosing from the simple relaxing routine by Include one to two of your favorite relaxing poses as part of your bedtime routine. Downward-facing dog is one yoga position that people often use when they need to relax and gently stretch their muscles. For a detailed walk-through of the downward-facing dog, check out the YouTube video by Yoga with Adriene entitled "Downward Dog – Downward Facing Dog Yoga Pose."

Conclusion

Many people view sleep as a time when they are completely unproductive, but as you have seen, this is far from the truth. When you are sleeping, your body is repairing itself and restoring necessary parts in more than a dozen separate processes. In fact, your body is just as active and productive at night as it is when you are awake. The only difference is the type of processes that occur.

You now know exactly what happens as you sleep, so you can better understand the importance of getting an optimum amount of sleep each night. Use the information presented throughout this book to give yourself the sleep you need. This will ensure that your body is properly rested and restored every twenty-four hours. You have also seen how the different stages of sleep affect your body. When you are getting enough restful sleep, it helps your entire life. You are more energized and productive during the day when you make sleep a priority. Increased productivity can help with everything from finding success at work, to getting good grades to being able to keep up with all of your social responsibilities.

When you do not get enough sleep, all aspects of your health can be affected, from stress affecting your mind and body to an increased risk of a number of health conditions. By noting the issues that affect you and reviewing your sleeping habits, you are in a good position to choose what will best help you gain sleep.

You also have learned about the major disorders that interfere with proper sleep and what you can do to address them. Not all sleeping problems are directly related to a medical condition. However, if they are, it is critical to get a prompt diagnosis so you can get started with treatment. The right treatment can help you sleep better and enjoy more productive days.

Sleep hygiene is also important. In many cases, a single change can make a huge difference in how you feel when you wake up in the morning. There are a host of natural remedies that can help you accomplish both appropriate sleep and alert wakefulness.

What you do during the day has an impact on your sleep. You now possess the tools you need to alter your daily routine so you can sleep well. These are relatively simple changes that you can start working on today. If you are not sleeping well right now, experimenting with these options may well help.

How you prepare for bed be the most important factor influencing your sleep. You now know exactly how a sleep routine can help and what you need to do to create one that helps you prepare for restful sleep.

Start today to create a bedtime routine. Choose one of the options listed in this book and start putting it into practice. Over the course of a week, add another one or two, until you have created a full thirty-minute pre-bed routine. After just a few days, you will start to notice positive changes in your ability to sleep. You can always make tweaks in the future if you need to change things up.

You now have all of the tools you need to be a more productive and efficient sleeper. So go ahead! Take the comprehensive information that is presented here and start putting it to work in your life. Keep in mind that you cannot change habits overnight. This is actually a good thing. Gradual change is better for your body and mind, because it allows you to adapt a little at a time. Taking your time also allows new habits to sink in and really work deeply into your life.

You can now look forward to a more restful and productive sleep. You can enjoy better energy during the day, fewer minor ailments, and better cognitive abilities. Welcome to your new journey toward a happier, healthier, and more rested you.

I hope this book was able to help you to learn more about sleep and what you need to do to get good sleep every night.

The next step is to put the information in this book into practice so you can start to improve your sleep right away. You can see the information in this book is the highly comprehensive, ensuring that you have the practical information you need to get effective sleep.

Finally, if you discovered at least one thing that has helped you or that you think would be beneficial to someone else, be sure to take a few seconds to easily post a quick positive review. As an author, your positive feedback is desperately needed. Your highly valuable five star reviews are like a river of golden joy flowing through a sunny forest of mighty trees and beautiful flowers! *To do your good deed in making the world a better place by helping others with your valuable insight, just leave a nice review.*

Thanks and Best of Luck

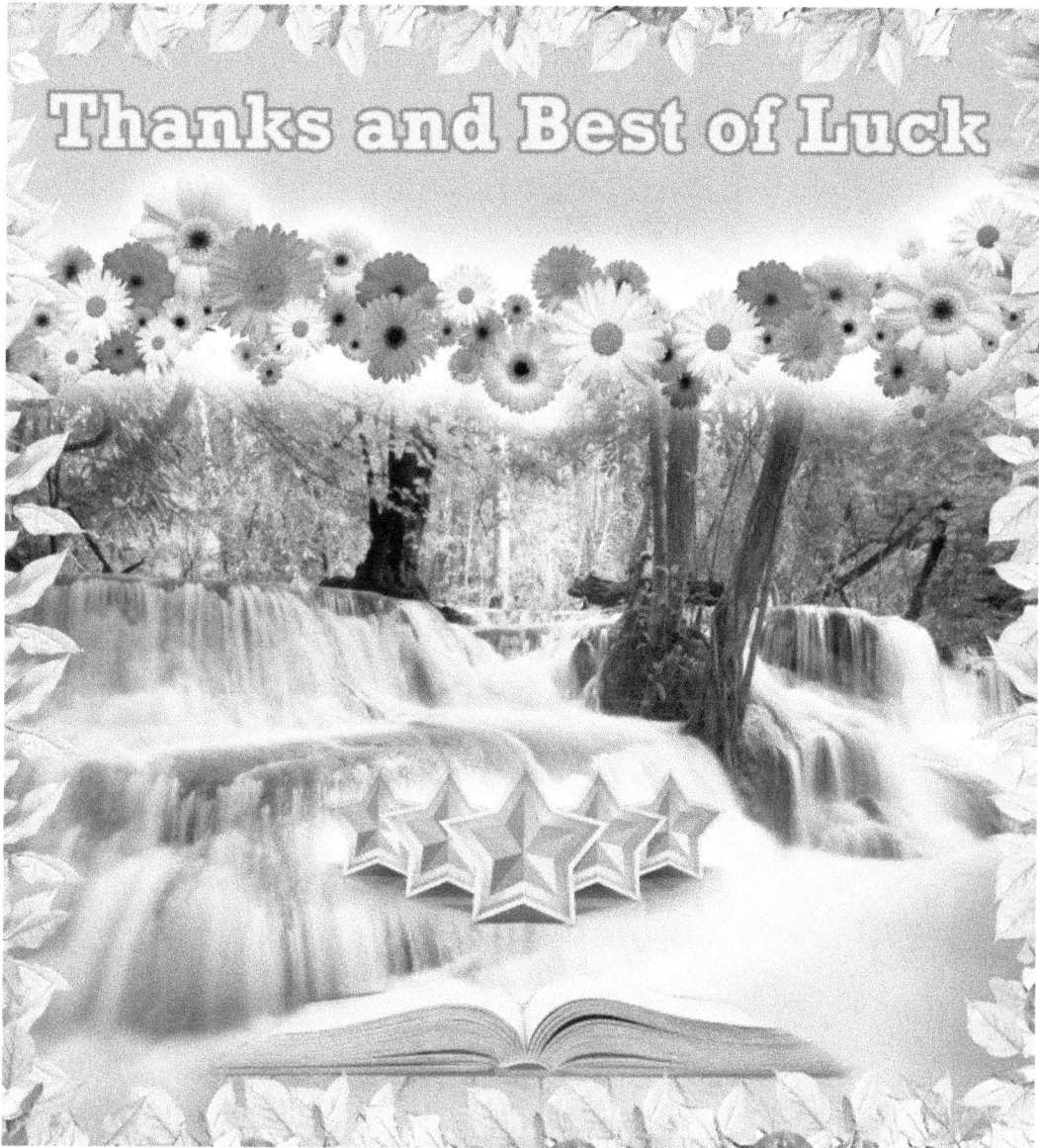

My Other Books and Audio Books
www.AcesEbooks.com

Health Books

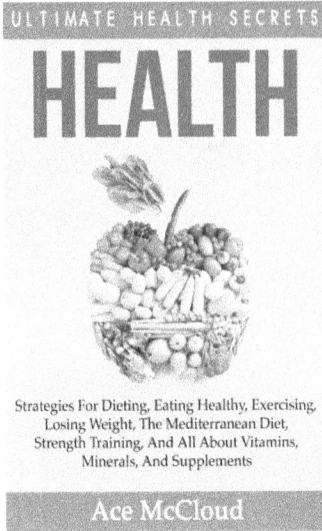

ULTIMATE HEALTH SECRETS

HEALTH

Strategies For Dieting, Eating Healthy, Exercising,
Losing Weight, The Mediterranean Diet,
Strength Training, And All About Vitamins,
Minerals, And Supplements

Ace McCloud

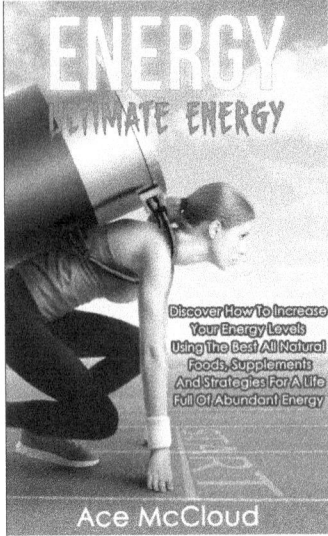

ENERGY
ULTIMATE ENERGY

Discover How To Increase
Your Energy Levels
Using The Best All Natural
Foods, Supplements
And Strategies For A Life
Full Of Abundant Energy

Ace McCloud

RECIPE BOOK

The Best Food Recipes
That Are Delicious, Healthy,
Great For Energy And Easy To Make

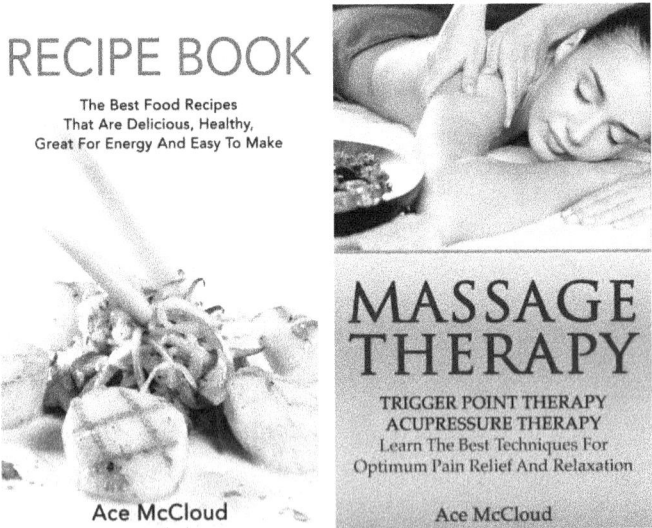

Ace McCloud

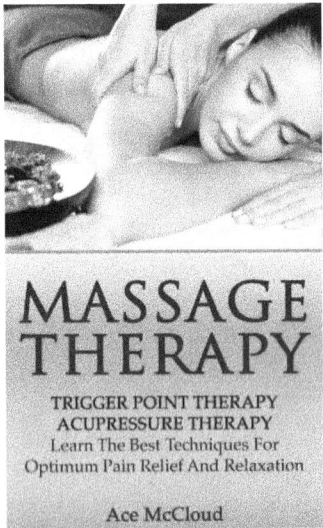

MASSAGE THERAPY

TRIGGER POINT THERAPY
ACUPRESSURE THERAPY
Learn The Best Techniques For
Optimum Pain Relief And Relaxation

Ace McCloud

LOSE WEIGHT

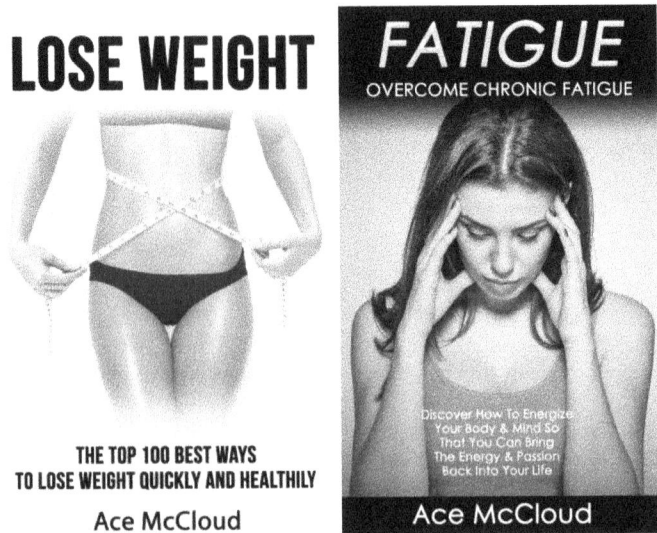

THE TOP 100 BEST WAYS
TO LOSE WEIGHT QUICKLY AND HEALTHILY

Ace McCloud

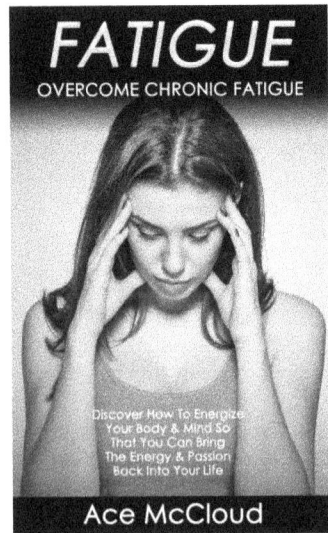

FATIGUE
OVERCOME CHRONIC FATIGUE

Discover How To Energize
Your Body & Mind So
That You Can Bring
The Energy & Passion
Back Into Your Life

Ace McCloud

Peak Performance Books

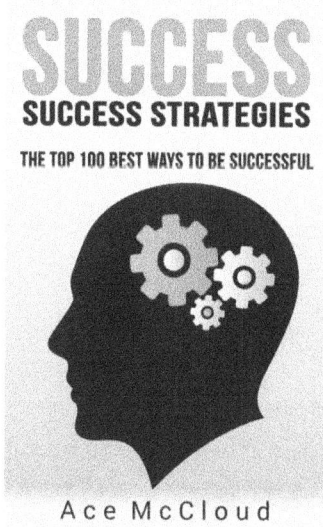

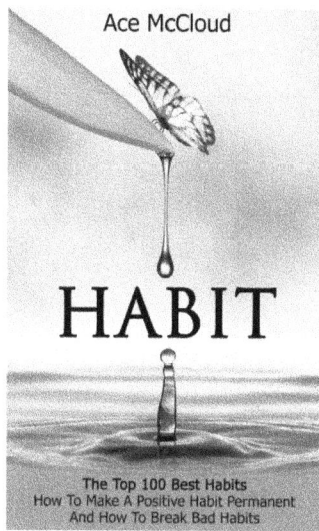

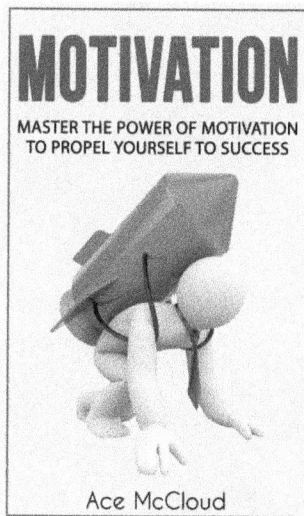

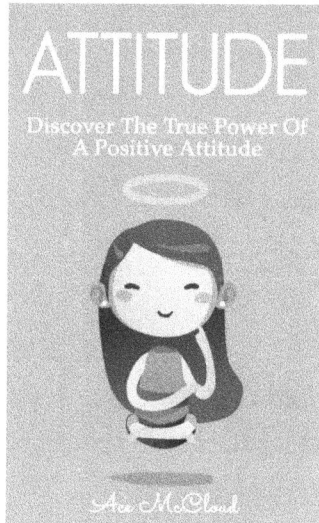

SUCCESS

SUCCESS STRATEGIES

THE TOP 100 BEST WAYS TO BE SUCCESSFUL

Ace McCloud

Ace McCloud

HABIT

The Top 100 Best Habits
How To Make A Positive Habit Permanent
And How To Break Bad Habits

MOTIVATION

MASTER THE POWER OF MOTIVATION
TO PROPEL YOURSELF TO SUCCESS

Ace McCloud

ATTITUDE

Discover The True Power Of
A Positive Attitude

Ace McCloud

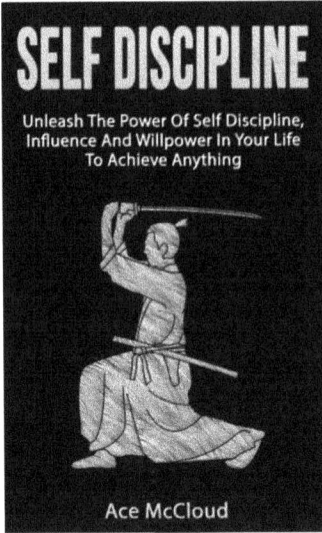

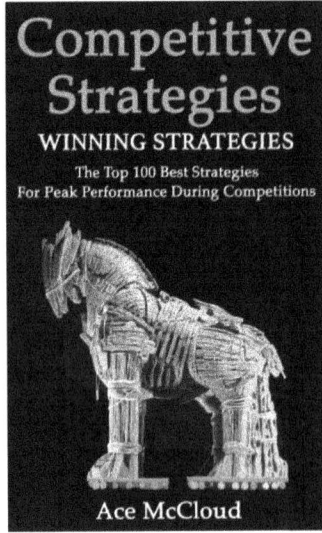

Be sure to check out my audio books as well!

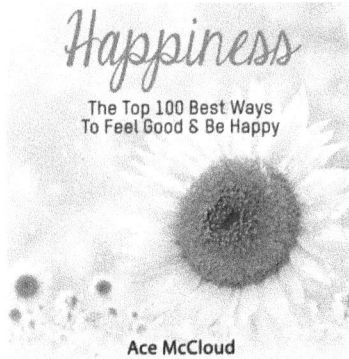

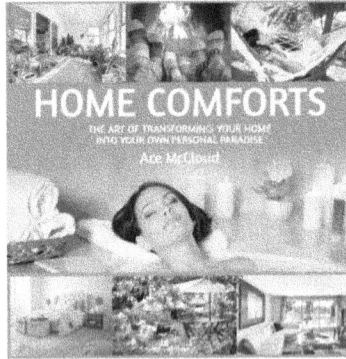

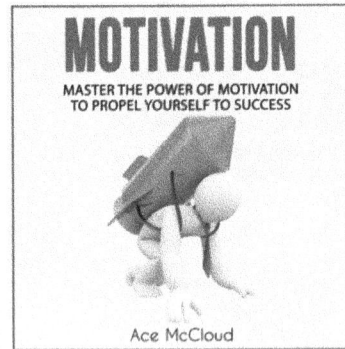

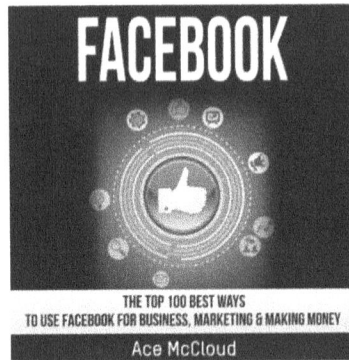

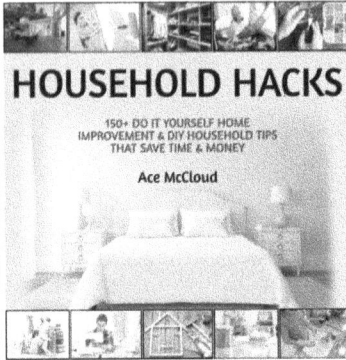

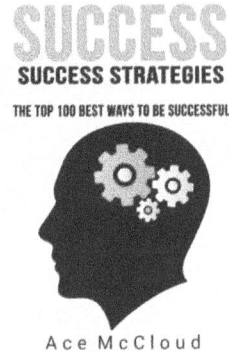

Check out my website at: **www.AcesEbooks.com** for a complete list of all of my books and high quality audio books. I enjoy bringing you the best knowledge in the world and wish you the best in using this information to make your journey through life better and more enjoyable! **Best of luck to you!**

www.ingramcontent.com/pod-product-compliance
Lightning Source LLC
Chambersburg PA
CBHW080630030426
42336CB00018B/3148